Chronic Fatigue Syndrome for Adults at 40:
Simple and Effective Ways to Treat CFS

Bella Kelvin

Table of Contents

I. Introduction

Chronic fatigue Syndrome (CFS) is a complicated illness defined by an intense, incapacitating weariness that does not improve with rest and is not caused by any underlying medical condition. The exhaustion can be so extreme that it interferes with everyday tasks, and patients may feel fully spent even after only a short period of exercise. Other symptoms of CFS include muscular discomfort, joint pain, headaches, sleep difficulties, and trouble concentrating and remembering.

The actual etiology of CFS is unclear, and there is no definitive diagnostic test for the condition at this time. However, evidence shows that a mix of variables, including viral infections, immunological malfunction, genetic susceptibility, and psychosocial stresses, may contribute to the development of CFS.

A patient must fulfill specific criteria defined by the Centers for Disease Control and Prevention (CDC) to be confirmed to have CFS. The prerequisites include a minimum of six months of detrimental fatigue that is not caused by a medical diagnosis, as well as at least four of the symptoms that follow: challenges with concentration or memory, a sore throat, tender lymph nodes, discomfort in the muscles, discomfort in the joints, headaches, unrefreshing sleep, and post-exertional malaise (a deteriorating of symptoms after physical or mental exertion).

CFS is a difficult illness to treat, and there is presently no cure. Treatment options, on the other hand, may include a mix of drugs, lifestyle modifications, and alternative therapies. Patients can additionally benefit from support groups and therapy to help them cope with the disorder's emotional toll.

It is critical to recognize that CFS is a valid medical disease that should be addressed seriously. Due to a lack of awareness regarding the condition, patients with CFS may confront suspicion and incredulity from healthcare practitioners, friends, and family members. Many individuals with CFS, however, may improve their symptoms and achieve a higher quality of life with the correct diagnosis and treatment.

Chronic Fatigue Syndrome (CFS) can be especially difficult for persons over 40 since it can worsen the physical and mental changes that come with aging. Below are some of the ways that CFS can impact adults over the age of 40:

- Reduced physical activity: CFS can induce extreme exhaustion, making it difficult for sufferers to do routine daily tasks including work, housework, and exercise. This can contribute to weight gain, muscle loss, and other health issues by leading to a more sedentary lifestyle.

- Discomfort and stiffness: Many individuals with CFS feel muscular and joint discomfort, which can worsen as they become older. This can make staying active even more difficult and lead to a more sedentary lifestyle, increasing the symptoms of CFS.

- Cognitive decline: CFS can cause issues with focus, memory, and cognitive function, which can be especially difficult for persons over 40, who may already be suffering age-related cognitive impairments. This can have an impact on professional performance, social relationships, and day-to-day activities.

- Other health problems: People with CFS may be more likely to acquire other health issues as they age, such as cardiovascular disease, diabetes, and osteoporosis. This might be attributed to decreased physical activity, inflammation, and other CFS-related problems.

- Emotional impact: Chronic fatigue syndrome (CFS) may be an extremely isolated and frustrating condition that can have a negative influence on a person's emotional well-being. This can be especially difficult for persons over the age of 40 who are dealing with other life transitions such as retirement, empty nests, and elderly parents.

Despite these obstacles, it's worth noting that many people with CFS can manage their symptoms and live productive lives. Many patients with CFS can improve their symptoms and achieve a higher quality of life with the correct diagnosis and treatment.

Stress and its impact on people over 40

Stress is a typical physical and psychological reaction to the demands and obstacles of life. It's how our bodies get ready for a threat or danger. Our bodies create stress chemicals like adrenaline and cortisol whenever we detect a threat, real or imagined. These hormones cause some physiological reactions that get our bodies ready to act, such as raising the heart rate, blood pressure, and breathing.

In moderation, stress may even be helpful since it keeps us attentive, motivated, and focused. For instance, a small bit of tension before a job interview might improve our performance by focusing and energizing us.

However, stress may harm our physical and emotional health if it persists or becomes excessive. Numerous health issues, such as anxiety, depression, sleeplessness, digestive issues, and cardiovascular disease, can be brought on by prolonged stress. Our immune system may be weakened as a result, leaving us more prone to sickness.

Numerous things, such as pressure at work, money troubles, relationship issues, health issues, and significant life transitions, can lead to stress. Each individual reacts to stress uniquely, so what is distressing for one person might not be for another. It's critical to identify your unique stress triggers and create appropriate coping mechanisms to deal with them.

Exercise, mindfulness, relaxation methods, time management, social support, and seeking professional assistance when necessary are all effective stress management strategies. We may improve our physical and mental health, our general well-being, and our capacity to deal with life's problems by successfully managing our stress.

People over 40 may be more affected by stress because of age-related changes and other aspects of their lives that may make them more susceptible to its physical and emotional consequences. The following are some effects that stress may have on adults over 40:

- Physical condition: Numerous physical health issues, such as high blood pressure, heart disease, diabetes, and obesity, can be attributed to chronic stress. Effective stress management is essential to preserving physical health because as people age, their chance of developing chronic disorders rises.
- Cognitive decline: Chronic stress has been associated with dementia and cognitive deterioration in older persons. The impact of

stress hormones on the cardiovascular system and the brain may contribute to this.

- Mental health: Anxiety, despair, and sleeplessness are just a few of the mental health issues that stress can contribute to. Due to age-related changes in brain chemistry and life events like retirement, losing loved ones, and financial worries, older persons may be more prone to these illnesses.

- Immune system: Long-term stress can impair immunity, leaving elderly people more prone to disease and infection. Given the higher risk of significant disease and consequences from COVID-19 for older persons, this can be especially worrisome.

Chronic stress may harm a person's general quality of life, making it more difficult to enjoy routine activities, maintain social connections, and discover meaning and purpose in life.

People over 40 can enhance their general health and well-being and lead more rewarding lives by adopting effective efforts to control their stress.

A summary of what readers may discover from the book is provided below:

Recognizing CFS: Readers will probably gain a thorough grasp of CFS, including its etiology, symptoms, and risk factors, from the book. It could help clarify how CFS differs from other ailments with similar symptomatology, such as fibromyalgia, and how it can affect a person's day-to-day activities.

Options for treating CFS: The book will probably go through a variety of CFS treatments, including both traditional and alternative therapy. It could include prescription drugs, dietary changes, lifestyle adjustments, and supplementary treatments like massage or acupuncture.

Techniques for managing stress: The book is likely to give readers a variety of efficient stress management methods that they may use to ease their tension and enhance their general well-being. These could consist of social support, exercise, time management, relaxation techniques, and mindfulness techniques. The book may also discuss the effects of stress on physical and mental health and provide readers with strategies for better stress management.

Modifications to one's lifestyle: The book may also offer readers pointers and advice on how to make quick changes to one's lifestyle that might lessen stress and enhance general health. This can entail altering one's eating habits, practicing good sleeping habits, and engaging in greater physical exercise each day.

In all, readers may anticipate learning in-depth information about CFS and stress, as well as useful tools and techniques for efficiently managing these disorders. Because of the book's apparent emphasis on simplicity and efficacy, it should be understandable and useful to readers from many walks of life.

II. Understanding CFS and Stress

Definition of CFS and its symptoms

The complicated and crippling disorder known as Chronic exhaustion Syndrome (CFS), also known as Myalgic Encephalomyelitis (ME), is defined by excessive exhaustion that lasts for at least six months and is not alleviated by rest. The following are some of the main signs of CFS:

- Excessive tiredness: Extreme weariness that is not eased by rest is the defining characteristic of CFS. This weariness may linger for weeks, months, or even years and may be so severe as to interfere with everyday tasks.

- Muscle and joint pain are common symptoms of CFS, and they can be quite painful and interfere with everyday tasks.

- Cognitive challenges: People with CFS may also struggle with cognitive challenges like memory, focus, and decision-making issues.

- Sleep problems: People with CFS typically have sleep disruptions, which can include trouble going to sleep, frequent nighttime awakenings, and a lack of wakefulness following sleep.

- Numerous CFS sufferers also endure regular headaches, which can be quite painful and incapacitating.
- Additional signs: People with CFS may also have a variety of additional symptoms in addition to these basic ones, such as nausea, sensitivity to light and sound, dizziness, and flu-like symptoms like fever and sore throat.

It's essential to remember that each person will experience CFS differently and that the disease is sometimes challenging to identify. It's vital to talk with your healthcare practitioner if you have chronic tiredness or other symptoms that are interfering with your daily life to identify the underlying reason and create an effective treatment plan.

Causes of CFS and its effect

Although the precise causes of Chronic Fatigue Syndrome (CFS) are not entirely understood, experts think that a mix of genetic, environmental, and behavioral factors is most likely to blame. The following are some of the most typical CFS causes and how they may impact adults over the age of 40:

- Infection with a virus: According to some experts, viral infections such as the Epstein-

Barr virus or human herpesvirus 6 may be the cause of CFS. Due to aging-related immune system changes that might make it harder for the body to fight off viruses, people over 40 may be more prone to certain diseases.

- Hormonal imbalances: The hypothalamic-pituitary-adrenal (HPA) axis, which controls the body's stress response, maybe a contributing factor in CFS. Age-related changes in the HPA axis may make persons more susceptible to developing CFS.

- Environmental toxins: Being exposed to environmental toxins, such as pesticides or heavy metals, may also make you more likely to have CFS. The likelihood that these poisons have built up in the bodies of those over 40 may be higher, raising their chance of getting CFS.

- Lifestyle variables: Poor food, inactivity, and long-term stress are a few lifestyle factors that might raise the chance of getting CFS. Due to changes in metabolism, muscle mass, and stress response that come with advancing age, those over 40 may be more susceptible to encountering these issues.

People over 40 may be more affected by CFS because they may be more susceptible to age-related changes in physical function and energy levels. Daily tasks might be complicated by CFS, making it challenging to work, care for loved ones, or take part in recreational activities. Additionally, it may result in sadness and social isolation, both of which can negatively affect general well-being.

Definition of stress and its impact

Stress is a normal reaction to pressure or stress, whether it be physical or emotional. It is a natural aspect of life and, in certain instances, it may encourage us to act or remain vigilant under trying circumstances. However, stress may significantly affect the body and psyche when it becomes overpowering or persistent.

The following are some physiological effects of stress on the body:

- Circulatory system: Chronic stress can elevate blood pressure and promote artery inflammation, which can increase the risk of heart disease.

- Digestive system: Stress can impair digestion and limit blood flow to the digestive tract, which can result in gastrointestinal issues including diarrhea, constipation, or stomach distress.
- Immune system: Long-term stress can impair immunity, making it more challenging for the body to fend against infections and diseases.
- Nervous system: Stress chemicals like cortisol and adrenaline, which impact the nervous system and induce symptoms like anxiety, irritability, and sleeplessness, can be released.

Some effects of stress on the mind include the following:

- Mood: Stress can cause changes in mood, including irritation, anxiety, or despair.
- Memory and concentration: Prolonged stress can impair memory and concentration, making it harder to concentrate or recall information.
- Behavior: Stress can cause behavioral changes, such as an increase in drug or

alcohol usage, binge eating, or social withdrawal.

- Mental health: Long-term stress might raise your chance of developing mental health issues including despair and anxiety.

In the end, stress may have a substantial negative effect on both the body and the mind, and long-term stress can result in a variety of physical and mental health issues. To preserve general well-being, it's crucial to successfully manage stress through approaches like exercise, mindfulness, and relaxation methods.

Causes of stress and its effect

Several variables might lead to stress, such as:

Stress at work: Those who have demanding professions, lengthy workweeks, or stressful work settings may be more susceptible to stress. People over 40 may be more prone to experiencing work-related stress since they may hold senior positions or have a heavier burden.

Stress in one's personal life can also be brought on by problems in one's relationships, finances, or role as a caregiver. Stress may be more common in those over 40 as a result of caring for elderly parents or worries about finances in preparation for retirement.

Health issues: Stress-producing chronic disorders or illnesses include those that interfere with everyday living or need extensive medical treatment. People over 40 may be more susceptible to chronic diseases or health problems.

Major life transitions: Stress can also be brought on by divorce, retiring, or losing a loved one. Those over 40 may be more prone to go through these difficult life transitions.

People over the age of 40 may have particularly severe consequences from stress because, due to physiological changes brought on by aging, they may be more prone to stress-related health problems. For instance, stress can raise the risk of heart disease, which already affects older persons more often. Age-related health problems like cognitive decline or osteoporosis can be made worse by stress.

Stress may also negatively affect mental health, and those over 40 may be more prone to depression, anxiety, or other stress-related mental health disorders. Effectively managing stress via practices like exercise, mindfulness, and relaxation methods can assist to reduce these effects and preserve general well-being.

III. Simple Ways to Treat CFS and Stress

Lifestyle changes

Making certain lifestyle adjustments can help you manage stress and CFS. The following adjustments may be helpful:

- Get adequate rest: Sleeping enough hours each night is crucial for controlling stress and CFS. Set a consistent sleep schedule and aim for 7-9 hours of sleep each night.
- Regular exercise might help you feel more energized and relieve stress. Starting with low-impact workouts like swimming, yoga, or walking can help you build up your stamina.
- Eat a balanced, healthy diet to support your overall health and energy levels. Eat a mix of fruits, vegetables, lean proteins, and healthy grains as your main focus.
- Use ways for reducing stress: Stress reduction and relaxation can be aided by

practices like yoga, deep breathing, and meditation.

- Practice stress-reduction methods: Methods like yoga, deep breathing, and meditation can help lower stress and encourage relaxation.
- Make self-care a priority. Making time for yourself may help you feel better and reduce stress. Examples include taking a soothing bath, reading a book, or spending time with loved ones.
- Manage your workload and responsibilities: Strive to strike a balance between the two, and refrain from taking on too much at once. Set tasks in order of importance and, where appropriate, assign work to others.
- Seek assistance: To help manage stress and mental health, think about joining a support group for CFS sufferers or speaking with a therapist or counselor.

Although these ways of living adjustments can help manage stress and CFS, it's vital to keep in mind that they may not be suitable for everyone.

The symptoms of CFS and stress can both be effectively managed with relaxation techniques. Here are some methods you might use:

Deep inhalation: Breath slowly and deeply through your nose, then exhale slowly through your mouth. Pay attention to how your breath feels as it enters and exits your body.

Progressive muscle relaxation: Contract and then relax every muscle in your body, beginning at the bottom and working your way up to the top.

Sit comfortably and practice mindfulness by concentrating on your breath. When your thoughts stray, simply bring them back.

Yoga: Practicing yoga can increase flexibility and strength while lowering stress.

Yoga-like movement and meditation are used in tai chi to encourage relaxation and lower tension.

Close your eyes and picture a tranquil, serene place, such as a beach or a forest.

Listen to a tape or participate in a guided imagery session to help you picture yourself in a serene, relaxing environment.

Take into consideration that everyone is unique, therefore not all relaxation techniques will be effective for you. Finding the methods that are most effective for you can need some trial and error. Additionally, even while these methods might be useful in controlling stress and CFS symptoms, they might not be viable alternatives to medical care. For the management of CFS, it's critical to design a specialized treatment plan in collaboration with a healthcare expert.

Alternative therapies

Numerous complementary and alternative therapies may be useful in controlling stress and CFS. Here are a few illustrations:

- Acupuncture: Thin needles are inserted into predetermined body locations during acupuncture treatments. It may be useful in lowering tension and discomfort since it is thought to assist regulate the energy flow in the body.
- Massage therapy: To encourage relaxation and relieve stress, muscles, and soft tissues are moved. It could be useful for controlling stress and CFS symptoms.
- Chiropractic treatment: To enhance function and lessen discomfort, chiropractic treatment includes manipulating the spine

and other joints. It could be useful for treating CFS symptoms including tiredness and discomfort.

- Herbal medications: Some herbal supplements, such as ginseng and ashwagandha, may be beneficial for boosting energy and lowering stress. Before ingesting any supplements, it's crucial to see a healthcare provider.
- Mind-body treatments: Mind-body treatments like hypnosis, biofeedback, and meditation can aid in promoting relaxation and lowering stress. They might be beneficial in treating CFS symptoms as well.

It's crucial to keep in mind that not all alternative therapies are suitable for everybody, and some might not even be supported by scientific research. Before experimenting with any alternative treatments, it's essential to consult a healthcare provider.

Medications and supplements

Many prescription drugs and dietary supplements have potential benefits for treating CFS and stress. Here are a few instances:

Antidepressants: Stress management and CFS management may both benefit from antidepressants. They function by bringing particular brain chemicals that impact mood into balance.

Anti-anxiety drugs: Anti-anxiety drugs may aid with stress and anxiety management. They function by lowering anxiety and soothing the neurological system.

Sleep aids: Sleep aids may be useful in treating insomnia, one of the symptoms of CFS. They function by encouraging sleep and minimizing nighttime vigilance.

Painkillers: Acetaminophen or ibuprofen are two painkillers that may be useful in treating CFS-related pain.

Supplements: Some supplements might be useful for controlling stress and CFS. For instance, melatonin and magnesium may be beneficial in fostering relaxation and enhancing sleep.

It's crucial to keep in mind that not all prescription drugs and dietary supplements are suitable for everyone and that some of them may have negative side effects or interact negatively with other drugs. Before ingesting any pharmaceuticals or dietary supplements, it's crucial to see a healthcare provider.

IV. Practical Tips and Strategies for Managing CFS and Stress

Daily habits and routines

Numerous everyday routines and behaviors might be beneficial in controlling stress and CFS. Here are a few instances:

- Get adequate rest: Getting enough sleep is essential for managing stress and CFS. Try to build a calming nighttime ritual and a regular sleep regimen.

- Regular exercise can help you manage stress and CFS, even though it may seem paradoxical. It's crucial, to begin with, low-impact exercises like stretching, yoga, or walking before progressively increasing the difficulty as acceptable.

- Eat a balanced diet: A nutritious diet can promote general health and help control the symptoms of CFS. A balanced diet should include enough fruits, vegetables, lean protein, and whole grains. Avoiding processed meals, alcohol, and caffeine may also be beneficial.

- Practice stress-reduction methods: Stress-reduction methods, such as progressive muscle relaxation, deep breathing, or meditation, can help you manage your stress and enhance your wellness.
- Prioritize tasks and control workload: To prevent exhaustion and overwork, tasks should be prioritized and the workload managed. Take pauses when necessary and divide work into small portions.
- Pace yourself: One of the most effective ways to control the symptoms of CFS is to pace oneself. This calls for segmenting tasks and preserving energy throughout the day.
- Ask for help: Asking for help from family, friends, or a healthcare provider can be beneficial in managing stress and CFS.

It's crucial to keep in mind that each person's experience with CFS and stress is different, and it could take some time to figure out what works best for them.

Building a support network is a crucial method for controlling CFS and stress. Here are some suggestions for developing a support network:

- Contact your family and friends: Share with your loved ones the nature of your illness and how it affects you. They might be a fantastic provider of emotional assistance.

- Join an advocacy group: Joining a support group may give you a feeling of belonging and link you with people who share your experiences. Online support groups are a fantastic alternative as well.

- Speak with a counselor: You can learn coping mechanisms from a therapist to control your stress levels and CFS symptoms. They may also offer you emotional support and aid in overcoming any challenging feelings you might be going through.

- Work with a medical expert: Your medical team can offer helpful support and direction for managing CFS symptoms. They can also assist you in determining any underlying medical issues that might be causing your exhaustion.

Self-care is something that you should do if you want to manage your CFS and stress. This might mean prioritizing your personal needs, taking breaks when necessary, and participating in activities you love.

Keep in mind that developing a support network is a lengthy and labor-intensive process. It's crucial to practice self-kindness and look for the tools and assistance you require to manage your illness.

How to balance work and personal life
When coping with CFS and stress, finding a balance between a job and personal life may be difficult. To establish balance, consider the following advice:

- Set reasonable objectives: It's critical, to be honest about your abilities and limitations. Avoid taking on more than you can handle and never be afraid to ask for assistance.
- Compile a schedule of your tasks and order them in order of importance to better manage your time. Don't be scared to delegate or let go of things that are less important, but rather, prioritize the chores that are most vital first.
- Take pauses: You may better control your energy levels and avoid burnout by taking

breaks throughout the day. Your workweek should include regular pauses that you may utilize to relax, meditate, or do other calming activities.

- Schedule your time: Scheduling your time might help you balance your personal and professional lives. Establish precise periods for work, rest, and leisure activities, and try your best to keep to them.

Talk to your employer about any modifications or accommodations that could be helpful if you're having trouble handling your job obligations. This might entail altering your workload or working hours, working from home, or taking time off if necessary.

Keep in mind that establishing balance requires time and effort. To properly manage your CFS and stress, it's crucial to be patient with yourself and give your needs a top priority.

V. Conclusion

Major importance of managing CFS and stress for people over 40

For adults over 40, managing CFS and stress is crucial for several reasons:

Keeping fit physically: Chronic weariness and stress may wear down the body and cause a variety of physical health issues. People over 40 can lower their chance of acquiring illnesses including heart disease, diabetes, and high blood pressure by controlling their CFS and stress.

Improving mental health: Prolonged stress and exhaustion can harm the mind, causing symptoms like anxiety, sadness, and mood swings. People over 40 can enhance their mental health and general well-being by controlling CFS and stress.

Increasing quality of life: It might be challenging to take pleasure in everyday activities and keep up social connections when you experience chronic weariness and stress. People over 40 can enhance their quality of life and participate more fully in their favorite activities by controlling these symptoms.

Taking steps to lessen the chance of burnout: People over 40 may have demanding employment, caregiving duties, or other pressures. They may lower their risk of burnout, retain their productivity, and be productive in both their personal and professional life by controlling their CFS and stress.

Slowing down the aging process: Prolonged stress and exhaustion have been shown to hasten age, causing premature sagging of the skin, hair, and body. People over 40 can slow down aging and enjoy a more youthful appearance and energy by controlling their CFS and stress.

To maintain their physical and mental health, improve their quality of life, and lower their risk of burnout and premature aging, persons over 40 must effectively manage their CFS and stress.

Things to Note:
Not by yourself: It can be difficult and alienating to deal with CFS and stress, but it's vital to keep in mind that you're not alone. There are services

available to help you and many other individuals who are dealing with these problems.

You don't need to drastically alter your lifestyle to manage CFS and stress; little changes can have a major impact. Small adjustments to your daily habits or the incorporation of relaxation methods can have a big influence on your well-being.

Asking for assistance is acceptable since managing CFS and stress can be difficult. You may handle these symptoms using a variety of tools, including talking to friends or family members, getting professional treatment, and joining support groups.

You should put your health and well-being first: As we become older, it becomes easier to put other obligations ahead of our health and well-being. But it's crucial to keep in mind that caring for oneself is necessary for our general quality of life. Setting your health and well-being as a top priority will help you better manage your CFS, reduce stress, and live a fuller life.

It's simple to feel trapped in a cycle of tension and exhaustion, but it's crucial to keep in mind that you are capable of making positive changes. You may manage CFS and stress and enhance your general well-being by taking action and putting the techniques described in this book into practice.

Remember that finding what works best for you when managing CFS and stress might take some time. The good news is that you may effectively control these symptoms and have a happier, healthier life by taking baby steps and being devoted to your health.

www.ingramcontent.com/pod-product-compliance
Lightning Source LLC
Chambersburg PA
CBHW061028250726
48659CB00020B/2344